# The Surgery Book

## 2022 EDITION

### Options and Explanations for Patients

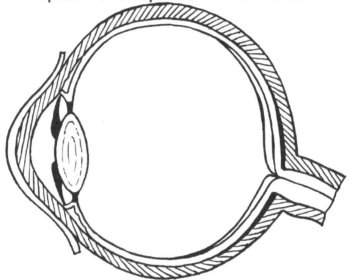

**David Woods MD**
**Robert Reeve MD**
**Edited by Phil Midling**
**This book is dedicated to**
**patients needing cataract surgery**

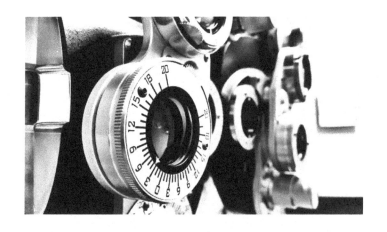

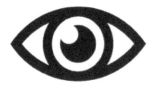

**The Risk and Reward of Cataract Surgery**
Our collective eyes have witnessed human history throughout the ages. They have seen the grandeur and splendor of life on earth, the skies and mountains and seas. Through the prism of our eyesight, we can detect the subtlest of movements, decipher vibrant and vivid color, and distinguish objects, shapes, and forms with exact and incremental precision.
Eyesight is one of our most cherished and valued senses. Our eyes are a window to our soul and our window to the world. Our collective vision has witnessed human history spanning the ages. We have seen the splendor and majesty of life here on

Earth —the skies and mountains and seas and observed our planet from space. Through the prism of our eyesight, we can detect the slightest and subtlest of movements, decipher vibrant and vivid color, and distinguish objects, shapes, and forms with exact and incremental precision.

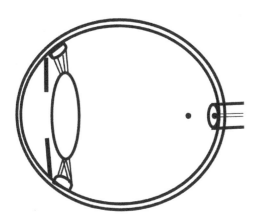

And yet, the eyes we are born are in a constant state of change and adjustment, besieged by the elements of that very same living environment, by the stress and strain of our daily life, and limited by our genetic makeup. It wasn't that long ago that we were essentially stuck with the vision hand we were dealt with at birth. But over the past half-century, modern advancements in technology have made it possible to not only improve eyesight but correct vision deficiencies and abnormalities that were once thought inoperable and incurable.

Ophthalmology and eye surgery for me was a natural choice as a career for me, after experiencing many times the potential for dramatic visual improvements in the lives of patients. Centuries of technological progress in science and eye surgery now allow patients and their surgeons to experience a transformative experience together. We hope to share the options from the surgeon's perspective in this book, so that an informed patient may obtain an optimized choice for their life.

Most cataract surgery patients are optimistic and for good reason. We have personally performed thousands of cataract surgeries in my career, including members of my own family, and the majority of those operations were qualitatively successful. And because of the success rate of such surgeries, many prospective patients expect perfect vision restored with little or no recovery time. And more often than not, this is the ultimate result. But, as with any surgery, there are potential complications. Cataract surgery has risk and can result in increased dry eye, irritation, pain, diminished focus, unexpected recovery issues, inflammation, and even loss of vision are possible. And that is the reason we are writing this book. To advise and educate prospective patients in their decision to undergo cataract surgery and improve their understanding of the overall risks and rewards of such surgery.

Over the past fifteen to thirty years as ophthalmologists, we have witnessed firsthand, the life-changing results of cataract surgery and

experienced with my patients the true joy that accompanies better and more useful vision.
In this book, we will be sharing not only my expertise based on education, training, and experience, along with objective and empirical evidence but also my subjective opinions as well. And those opinions may very well differ from the opinions of other medical experts in my field. And that's okay. Just as every eye is different, the perspective through which we observe is equally different, unique, and subjective.

**RISK: Improving Outcomes & Comments on Risk**

Even the most skilled and cautious of surgeons encounters potential and various complications: Everything from a piece of cataract being left behind to the occurrence of rare infections. One of the most proficient surgeons known, Dr. Takayuki Akahoshi of Japan, reported (private conference report) 29 infections in 300,000 cases. That is approximately one infection for every 10 thousand surgeries. Remarkably low, but not zero. Most surgeons don't have a volume of 300,000 surgeries, remarkable, and my tribute to pioneers such as Dr. Akahoshi for their safety and efficiency record. Impacting human lives for good is the goal of this now worldwide surgical endeavor.

**Basic Eye Anatomy**

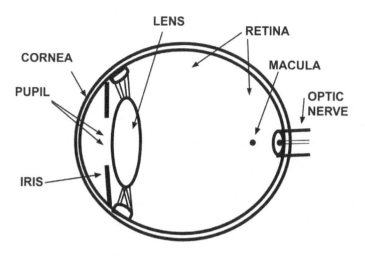

## ANATOMY OF THE EYE

**Light travels through:**

**The Cornea:** a clear layer in front of the eye. Often operated on for LASIK (Laser In Situ Keratomilieusis). Incisions are made on the cornea to do cataract surgery inside the eye.

**Anterior Chamber:** between the cornea and iris/lens. It is filled with aqueous fluid. The anterior chamber is the site of removal of cataract pieces during cataract surgery.

**The Iris:** The colored part of our eye. It is dilated for cataract surgery, enlarging the pupil.

**The Lens:** a protein crystalline-filled structure, encapsulated by an elastic sac. It functions to focus light, separate the aqueous-filled anterior chamber from the vitreous-filled posterior chamber. Cataracts are a cloudiness of the proteins inside the crystalline lens. Light rays cannot focus properly through cloudy cataracts, and so

**Vitreous:** protein strands that are mostly clear and fill the posterior chamber of the eye. Vitreous has attachments to the retinal periphery.

**Macula:** the central visual focus area for fine detail vision, small print, and the most specialized part of the retina. A healthy macula contributes to good vision. A disease of the macula may have vision loss in the center of vision.

**Retina:** The neurologic tissue that receives light, and processes a signal to the brain for vision. Its neuron layers are light-sensitive and its fibers contribute to form the optic nerve.

**Optic Nerve:** A large nerve tract carrying visual information from the eye to the brain for processing. A damaged optic nerve will reduce vision, such as in advanced glaucoma, or ischemic optic nerve damage (optic neuropathy).

**What is a Cataract?**

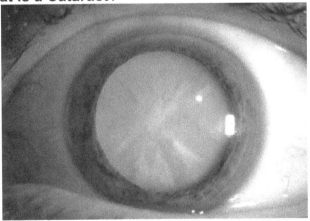

**A 'cataract', cloudy lens, with a 'waterfall' type appearance in the pupil**

A cataract is a 'cloudy' lens inside the eye. The word 'cataract' means 'waterfall' and is derived from the pearly appearance in the pupil of an advanced cataract. Perhaps you have seen the grey pupil of an older pet dog, with a pearly white appearance replacing a normal dark pupil. A human lens rests behind the pupil of the eye and functions to focus light onto the retina, much like an old-style camera that has a lens to focus light on the film of the camera. The "film" inside a human eye, that captures images and transmits them electrically through nerve fibers, is the retina. The retina has a central area that receives the focused light, and is the most sensitive part for small detail vision, and is called the macula.

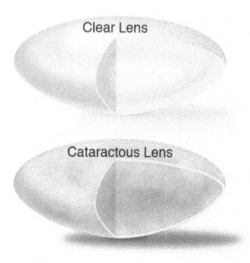

**The opacity of the human lens causes cloudiness and visual decline**

The human eye needs a clear lens to see properly. Light rays contribute to clear images when they converge to a single point. The human lens does this well when it's clear, and creates blurry and glary images when the lens is cloudy. Imagine looking through a frosted glass window pane or a darkened glass, the vision is reduced constantly.

Images focused on the macula, travel by electric signal along the nerve fibers of the optic nerve. The optic nerve consists of a bundle of a million small nerve fibers, each providing some image from a part of the retina, through nerve conduction, to the brain for visual processing. The optic nerve passes into the brain and eventually passes this information along, to make sense of the images.

The eyes' natural ability to focus light on the retina depends on having a clear lens. If it turns cloudy, light is scattered and images portrayed to the human brain are blurry or cloudy images.

The human lens is typically born with clear onion-like layers of cells filled with crystalline protein. It is encapsulated by an elastic-like sack called the "capsular bag", or the lens capsule. This capsule is suspended behind our pupil by tiny fibers called zonules, holding the lens securely like springs around a trampoline.

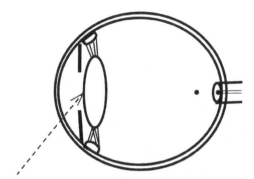

**The HUMAN LENS at BIRTH is CLEAR**

Think of the human lens like an M&M piece of candy. The candy shell is like the capsular bag, and inside the M&M are a peanut and chocolate layer, like the nucleus and cortex of the lens (lenticular cells filled with crystalline protein).

The human lens has no blood supply directly. There are no capillaries or blood vessels to it directly. The lens receives nourishment, glucose, oxygen, and other nutrients it needs by absorption from the fluid around it. The lens protein-filled clear cells have very slow growth over decades of human life. It's no wonder cataracts develop from age alone, as the cells eventually get more compact, stiff, and dense, with increased cloudiness changing the transparency of the lens.

A cataract is a cloudy lens inside the eye. A cloudy lens will not focus light as sharply, brightly colored images, or with less glare than a clear lens.

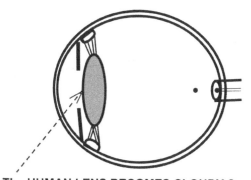

**The HUMAN LENS BECOMES CLOUDY &
BLURRY WITH A CATARACT**

The scattered light is often observed by patients as glare and visual blur. This can interfere with night driving, rain and headlight glare, sun glare. Smaller details may be harder to discriminate and work with small print or reading may become slower and more challenging.

A cataract shown here is evidenced by the yellowish/green discoloration in the patients' pupil. Thousands of years of discovery and recent decades with leaps in technology now allow surgery for cataract removal and placement of an artificial lens implant that is more clear, and many times with better focus, than a cloudy cataract. We will discuss many of the benefits and risks of cataract surgery and their implications, options, and context for cataract surgery today.

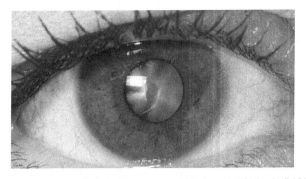

## Who Invented Cataract Surgery?

For much of human history, cataracts were removed by a technique referred to as "Couching." Couching is the process of moving a dense cloudy lens from the pupil and visual pathway inside the eye, bypassing a needle or instrument inside the eye, and simply dislodging it out of the pupil.

Couching was the primitive surgical method used in Egypt, Asia, and the historical world for approximately 2000 years. Though leaving the cataractous lens inside the eye, displaced into the vitreous cavity, was not always an ideal situation. Couching did offer some improvement and was a better alternative than living with a completely clouded cataract. And even then, a patient's vision focus was in a permanently deteriorated state. When glasses were eventually invented, patients still needed very thick lenses to compensate for their dysfunctional natural lenses. Think "Coke bottle" glasses. These thick glasses for the absence of a functional lens in the eye were called "aphakic spectacles".

Cataract surgery was first revolutionized in Europe in the 1800s when the dense cloudy cataract was removed by surgery. The aseptic surgical technique allowed "Lens Extraction" to be born with some safety. No longer would a rock-hard cataract float aimlessly through the back of the eye causing problems like high eye pressure and retinal damage.

Fast forward to World War II. A young British surgeon named Harold Ridley was on duty when he treated Mouse Cleaver, a pilot whose fighter plane cockpit shield had exploded causing shards of pyrex to become embedded into the pilot's eyes. The pyrex did not inflame the eye.

Dr. Ridley successfully proposed and demonstrated that lens implants inside the eye could be inert and nonreactive to the immune system of the body. He was later knighted by the Queen of England and awarded a Nobel prize for his efforts, restoring more useful vision to millions of people and soon to be billions with the advent of lens implant cataract surgery, or intraocular lens implants (abbreviated as IOL's).

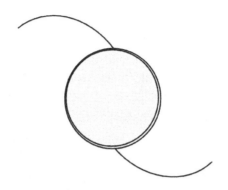

**An Intraocular Lens Implant**

**A CHRONOLOGY OF MODERN CATARACT SURGERY**

**1950** - Harold Ridley implants first Intraocular Lens in WWII pilot Mouse Cleaver. Ridley was later awarded the Nobel Prize and knighted by Queen Elizabeth.

**1960s** - Intraocular Lens Implants (IOL's) Improve

**1970s** - Incisions & Lens Extraction Improve, lowering risks of glaucoma, retinal detachment, and blindness.

**1980s** - Safety & Visual Outcomes Improve with standardizing of "in the capsular bag" Lens Implants

**1990s** - LASIK & Laser Vision Correction Occurs, and Cataract Surgery also improves visual focus outcomes

**2000s** - Multifocal Lens Implants and Astigmatism Controlling IOL's become available (Premium Lens Implants)

**2010s** - Multifocal Lenses that also help control Astigmatism become available (MFIOL's with astigmatism control). The femtosecond laser is available.  Micro-implants for glaucoma control arrive and improve significantly to lower eye pressure.

**2020**  - Trifocal lens implant arrives.

2021 - The Light Adjustable Lens arrives   (the first adjustable
        focus IOL after surgery once it is implanted)

## Who gets Cataracts?

Most likely all of us will get cataracts if we live long enough. Consider it part of successful aging. Cataracts usually are well underway and developing by the time we reach our seventieth birthday. It may occur earlier if we have experienced trauma, diabetes, a family history of early cataracts, various medical conditions with inflammatory disorders, poor nutrition, past smoking, or other risk factors.

## Symptoms of Cataracts

Symptoms of cataracts can include cloudy vision, glare symptoms with night glare, headlights, sunlight glare, blurry vision, and reading and driving difficulty.

Cataracts will often shift the focus of the eye, or refractive shifts, that alter one's glasses prescription. This may prompt more visits to the eye doctor to "update glasses" more often. One may "chase the cataract" and update glasses several times to get better focus, but ultimately refractive shifts often indicate cataract changes are significantly underway and time is approaching for potential cataract removal. A doctor's advice helps prepare risks, benefits, and options.

## How is cataract surgery performed?

Cataract surgery today is routinely performed as a minor procedure under intravenous anesthesia or I.V sedation. The comfort of intravenous sedation is helpful to the patient, and also to the surgeon. A relaxed and comfortable patient assists surgery to be an easier process.

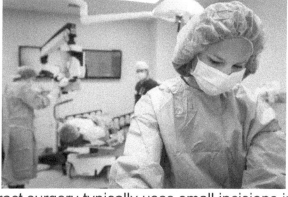

Cataract surgery typically uses small incisions in the peripheral cornea, and using a surgical microscope, the surgeon breaks up and removes the cloudy lens. The capsular bag is retained to hold in place a clear lens implant, which is unfolded through the small incision using an IOL injector (intraocular lens injector). The special instrumentation used through the small incisions to break up and remove the cataract is a special ultrasound aspiration instrument called phacoemulsification, or 'Phaco'. Sedation is administered through intravenous sedatives (IV sedation) to assist relaxation during the surgery. Sedation may be light, moderate, or deep. Often the comfort of the patient is the goal and so some patients may be aware, yet comfortable, for the procedure. Patients naive to relaxing medications, alcohol, and pain meds often fall asleep with sedation. The anesthesia provider has a goal of comfort for the patient and allowing breathing and the airway of the patient to be safe, as patients typically breathe on their own during this procedure.

Patients are not paralyzed or intubated for a general anesthetic due to an increased risk of such anesthesia for cataract surgery. General anesthesia causes paralysis and increases stress on the heart, lungs, and the risk of an adverse event. Intubation can be done for cataract surgery but this is usually limited to those with severe mental disability to understand the prerogative to remain still during surgery.

Deep anesthesia with IV sedation is possible and an option for some patients, helping spare the need for intubation, in cases where cooperation is limited during surgery. Ultimately it is a judgment call based on the estimation of risk by the anesthesia provider and the surgeon. These decisions are a balance of the surgeon's experience, the complexity of the case, the medical risk of deep sedation and intubation.

In my experience, topical anesthetic eye drops and anesthetic medications are applied inside the eye to alleviate pain and provide anesthesia during surgery. Blood pressure, heart rate, and oxygen are monitored by an anesthesia provider.

The procedure is often done without the use of sutures and the resulting incisions are sealed with hydration of saline and pressurizing the eye. Antibiotics and anti-inflammatory injections may be administered. Patients are frequently able to resume normal activities within one week to two weeks.

**Cataract Surgery Planning**
**Before surgery:**
1. Consultation with the cataract surgeon.
   - Discuss indications, goals, and risks of surgery
   - Evaluate candidacy to have cataract removal
   - Present options for surgery, such as goals for focus
   - Discuss risks, including the risk of complications, failure to improve vision, risks of glasses, dryness, pain, more surgery.
2. Measurements of the eye.
   - Ultrasound optical biometry is performed to measure the eye length and the curvature of the cornea. These measurements are used to calculate a lens implant power that is selected for the surgery.
3. Fasting on the day of surgery ...
   - You should typically not eat or drink anything for 8 hours before surgery. Most centers inform you to eat or drink nothing after midnight for this reason (NPO after midnight, or nothing by mouth).

**The architecture of the surgery**
Cataract surgery has several steps inside the Operating Room:

1. Prep and drape the patient in a sterile fashion
   - Recline the patient in a supine fashion
   - Place IV, blood pressure cuff, oxygen, and cardiac monitors
2. Surgical Incisions.
   - We typically place a 2.2 mm temporal corneal incision and a 1 mm clear corneal incision a few clock hours away from the main incision.
3. Stabilize the anterior chamber with viscoelastic.
   - Viscoelastic is a gelatinous material that is bio-compatible as it's composed of elongated proteins to form a clear gel.
4. Circularly open the capsule to reveal the cataract.
5. Dissect the capsule from the cataract by applying saline through a small syringe and cannula. The lens nucleus and cortex then spin freely.
6. Divide the cataract into pieces and remove and aspirate the pieces using phacoemulsification.
7. Polish the capsule by removing all cortex using a special irrigation/aspiration handpiece (the I/A handpiece) on all cortex adherent to the inside aspect of the capsular bag.
8. Fill the capsular bag with viscoelastic and then place the intraocular lens in the capsular bag.
9. Remove all the viscoelastic in the eye with the I/A handpiece.
   - Place antibiotic injection inside the eye for prevention of infection, and a cortisone-type injection of Kenalog under the eyelid inside the conjunctiva, to prevent inflammation and edema of the retina.

10. Seal the corneal sutures with saline irrigation so that they are watertight with no leaks. Place drops of antibiotic and/or iodine on the eye to further prevent infection.

This is the basic procedure for me at this time. It's changing in subtle ways all the time. If extra steps are being done for astigmatism control, such as the femtosecond laser or a toric lens implant, then the surgery will vary.

A lens implant is 5 to 6 millimeters typically in the width of the central portion (the 'optic'), with small arms or haptics as they are called, which stabilize the lens in the capsular bag in mid-pupil to assist focus.

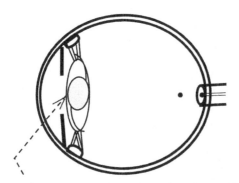

INTRAOCULAR LENS IMPLANT (IOL)

## What is an Intraocular Lens Implant (IOL)

Cataract surgery involves the removal of the cloudy lens and replacing it with an artificial lens implant called an Intraocular Lens or IOL. Pseudophakia is the condition of having one's lens replaced, the Latin term for an artificial lens is 'pseudophakia'.

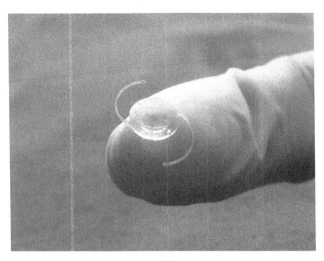

Cataract surgery in the United States has greatly evolved as a medical procedure over the past twenty years. New lens implant technology has facilitated the improvement of focus over the past few decades.

.

The implantation of an artificial lens implant occurs through a small incision in the cornea, usually less than 2.7 mm in size.

The lens implant is about 6 mm in size for the optic or central focus portion of the lens and 11 mm for the small arms, or haptics, that maintain centration of the lens implant.

The clear capsular bag which holds the lens implant is human tissue, which is preserved when the cataract is removed. The capsular bag is a 9-micron thick elastic tissue capsular sack.

Thank goodness for excellent microscopes that make operating on this clear, thin, fragile capsular sack possible.

The lens implant is "unfolded" as it is inserted through the small incision, and the small haptics press inside the capsular bag to keep the optic centered securely in the patients' pupil.

A well-centered lens implant occurs when the haptics push against the capsular bag. The bag itself is held in place anatomically by zonules, which are many small dense fibers that pull on the capsule radially, like the springs pulling on a trampoline tarp tightly. These small ropy fibers remind me of Spider Man's webbing, pulling on the sac to keep it in place.

## What types of Intraocular Lens Implants are available?

Lens Implants available for routine cataract surgery are:

1. **Standard** Lens Implant, or the Monofocal Lens Implant.
2. **Toric** Lens Implant for Astigmatism control
3. **Multifocal** Lens Implant
4. **Multifocal** Lens Implant that also has **Astigmatism** Control.

### Pick the Lens that is Best for You

Standard Lens:  Least Cost, single focus, use glasses

- Consider distance or near goal of focus after surgery  carefully as it only has a single focus
- Glasses may still be required.
- No additional cost for the lens

Standard Monofocal Lens Implant:

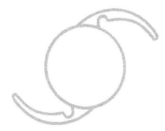

Toric Lens or Femtolaser: Correct astigmatism & sharpen focus
- Distance or near focus decision
- Glasses may still be required
- Extra cost

Toric Monofocal Lens Implant:

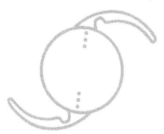

Multifocal Lens & Femtolaser:  Least need for glasses
- Panoptix (trifocal) or ActiveFocus +2.50 lens (bifocal with less glare) also with less near
- Glasses may still be required
- Extra cost

Multifocal Lens Implant (Toric version is shown here):

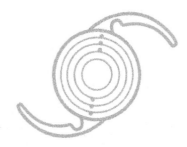

We will discuss each of these in the following sections in more detail.

In the United States, insurances will cover costs for the standard or monofocal lens implant, but additional costs are not typically covered for the specialty lens implants of the toric and multifocal lenses. The specialty lenses are considered elective not medically necessary. Therefore special treatments to reduce dependence on glasses are additional costs to patients.

**The Standard Monofocal IOL**

Lens Implants can be standard monofocal lens implants (most common), Toric Lens implants that may assist to reduce astigmatism, Multifocal lens implants, that provide a range of vision, and Toric Multifocal lens implants, that provide a range of vision and may assist to reduce astigmatism. Accuracy for better lens implants to correct focus and decrease blur from oval-shaped eyes now exists, called astigmatism correcting toric lens implants.

The standard IOL (Intraocular Lens) is by far the most commonly used IOL in the United States. The standard lens has a single focal point. It requires usually no extra out-of-pocket cost. Most patients are expected to require glasses to fine-tune vision and provide any range of vision they lack. Most patients choose to optimize distance focus with a standard lens in both eyes.

**Monovision** (1 eye with distance, 1 eye with near focus without glasses on) is an option with the Standard IOL.

A Standard Monofocal IOL does not always have to be focused on distance.

## 2. "Toric" Monofocal Lens Implant, or "Astigmatism Correcting" Lens Implant.

The use of this lens is used to improve the focus of the eye for patients that have an oval-shaped cornea. The lens implant must be aligned inside the eye to improve focus with the direction of existing astigmatism in the patient. There is an estimated 20 percent chance however that the patient will still be required to use glasses based on FDA trials, or in other words, an 80 percent chance good focus without glasses is achieved using a Toric lens implant. Since the lens is monofocal, or "single focus", it does not provide a range of vision. It is a single focus, and the patient must also decide if near or distance sight is to be optimized. Glasses are typically used to provide a range of vision otherwise. And yes, a nearsighted patient who chooses distance will lose near vision. Almost any patient could choose to have near vision after surgery but typically most do not.

**Monovision** (1 eye with distance, 1 eye with near focus without glasses on) is an option with the Toric IOL.

A Toric IOL does not always have to be focused on distance.

A **Toric** IOL may choose which focal point is being optimized .. distance, mid-range (about 20 inches), or near focus (about 15" from the eye).

3. **Multifocal** Lens Implant.

 Using special IOL manufacturing technology, the Multifocal Lens is a distance lens implant that can provide a range of both near and distance focus. This lens creates both a near image and a distance image on the retina, providing multifocality. Some risks of these lenses include out-of-pocket costs, about a 10% chance of still requiring glasses, and the appearance of halos or circular glow around lights, especially at night or with headlights.

**More on Multifocal Lens Implants**

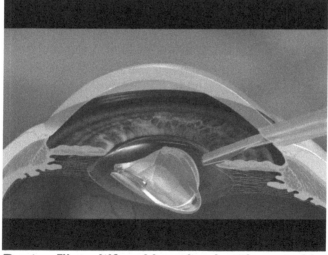

**a Restor ™ multifocal lens implant inserted into the capsular bag**

Multifocal Lens Implants have been improving since their first approval in the United States in 2005. The purpose of these lenses is to attempt to restore near and distance vision simultaneously in each eye. The technology is an additional tool to expand the range of vision and help reduce dependence on spectacles in many cases.

This technology has advantages but, as in all medical procedures, has limitations as well. The most common type of multifocal lens uses diffraction, the splitting of light rays to two focal points. This is accomplished with diffractive rings on the surface of the lens implant, such as the Alcon Pantoptix Trifocal IOL, the Alcon Restor Active Focus multifocal IOL, and the Johnson & Johnson Tecnis Multifocal IOL.

The best candidates for this procedure are those who desire to improve upon their visual range and reduce the use of glasses. Such patients accept the fact that they may not be able to read small print or drive at night as well as they used to. Even with this procedure, however, ten to twenty percent of patients still end up requiring glasses according to FDA studies. The fact that 80-90% of patients with multifocal lens implants are glasses-free is encouraging that technology is improving.

Patients who may not be ideal candidates for this procedure include those with eye medical conditions such as severe glaucoma or macular degeneration, those with high demand visual needs, perfectionist expectations, or those who simply desire glasses.

**Panoptix and ReStor Multi-Focal Lens Implants: Near and distance vision**

Multifocal lens implants, including the Panoptix, ReStor, and Tecnis Multifocal lens implants, provide useful near and distance vision with less dependency on the need for spectacles. Again, results can vary and potential candidacy should be individually determined and discussed with a physician.

Multifocal lens implants provide an improved range of vision and have allowed eye surgeons to correct both near and distance vision to a finer degree than ever before. The implantation and prescription of these lenses require a complete medical eye examination to determine candidacy and fit for lifestyle as well as consultation to discuss the risks, benefits, and overall prognosis for success.

Patients' expectations can still exceed technology, however, as this is not one's birth lens, and room for improvements in the technology still occur (See more discussion later in this book on Multifocal lens implants).

**The Light Adjustable Lens by RXSight**

The Light Adjustable Lens (LAL) has been in developemnt since early 2005. Dr. Dan Schwarz came to UC Davis and presented an incredible technology where the lens implant could be modified after implantation into the eye, and fine-tune or adjust, or sharpen the visual focus for patients. The theoretical benefits are, you never know exactly what the focus would be after surgery, but if you can fine tune the visual focus after implantation, then benefits for sharper vision could go up. Well, it's now 2022 and we are implanting the LAL and doing the adjustments with RXSight's Light Delivery Device (the LDD). The LDD is used to apply UV light to the LAL inside the eye. About 60 to 90 seconds of treatment will be utlizied to adjust the focus of the IOL. After one or two of these adjustments, another set of treatments are done to "Lock-In" the focus of the LAL. That means the LAL will no longer be adjustable or responsive to UV light. Patients in 2022 are required by the FDA and their labeling to protect their eyes from exposure to UV light after surgery and until about 3 to 4 weeks after surgery when the final lock-in treatment is performed. After this lock-in, the visual focus is no longer adjustable, and the special UV-blocking glasses worn indoors and outdoors after surgery, are no longer needed. It is recommended to do both eyes with the LAL one week apart or so, so that the use of the UV glasses, the adjustment treatments (one or two visits usually), and the lock-in treatment (usually two visits and treatments) are done on both eyes simultaneously. Otherwise, it becomes a lot of visits to the eye doctor!

**The Light Adjustable Lens is a single focus lens**
The Light Adjustable Lens is essentially a single focus lens. But, it has the advantages of correcting for small to moderate, to even higher amounts of astigmatism that remain after surgery. The "adjustability" for residual refractive error is limited to about 3.5 diopters of myopia or hyperopia, and about 3.5 diopters of astigmatism. This is

significant, as many patients have already corrected a highly myopic or highly hyperopic prescription at the moment of their new lens implantation (the surgeon will pick the lens power that has the best focus calculated), and then the light is able to be adjusted for focus even further.

The benefits of the LAL are becoming clearer with more experience. Some patients have had prior corneal surgery, such as LASIK, PRK (photorefractive keratectomy), or RK (Radial Keratotomy) increasing the "noise" around surgery calculations. They have corneas that are not mathematically as simple as a pristine cornea. Even the newest generation of lens implant biometry machines makes assumptions of corneal shape in the IOL calculation. The optimism surrounding LAL is an improved opportunity to adjust focus after surgery for these types of measurement issues. The patient themselves will have an opportunity to "try the vision" with trial lens glasses and determine if that is an improvement of the focus they are experiencing, or lock-in the visual focus as acheived. These are exciting times in eye care and cataract visual outcomes.

Stability of the prescription is often a question. What will happen in 1 year? 3 years? 5 years? Will I be back in glasses for distance. The answer is not uniformly the same for everyone. If you have been stable with little fluctuation in glasses for decades, you will probably not experience much fluctuation. If you needed to update your glasses every year or two, then you may continue to have

30

fluctuations in your distance focus after surgery. Removing the cataract removes the most highly fluctuating component of the glasses prescription in the anatomy of the eye, but the final lens position, and the corneal shape of people do show some people that fluctuate in their focus more than others.

The visual outcomes are 96% of patients with the LAL are 20/30 or better with uncorrected vision. 72% of patients are 20/20 with their uncorrected vision. These are useful guidelines for patients for comparison to other options for the refractive cataract surgery procedure.

**Could the LAL be used to target Monovision?**
Yes. As a single focus lens implant, monovision is a very good option for many LAL patients. It's probably best for all parties if a person has experienced monovision by previous contact lens trials, prior to locking-in a monovision visual setup. We will explore review more about the zones of visual performance, monovision

**The Zones of Vision**
**Focus & Range of vision when not wearing glasses after surgery**

| Zone 1 (Far) | Zone 2 (Mid-Range) | Zone 3 (Near) |
|---|---|---|
| Greater than 36 inches away | About 20 inches from eyes | About 15 inches from eyes |

| T.V. | Computer | Phonebook |
|---|---|---|
| Night Driving | Cooking | Smart Phone |
| Road Signs | Grocery Shelf | Make-up |
| Movies    Golf | Newsprint | Small Print |

A monofocal standard lens implant, or a toric monofocal lens implant, has a single focal point unless a person is wearing glasses to give them both near and far focus. A single focus, e.g. monofocal, lens implant can be set for near or far focus. Hence 2 eyes set for distance focus requires reading glasses, and two eyes set for near focus will require distance glasses. The functional zones used for guiding decisions are listed above.

Understanding which patients have accustomed to which zones already, and which zone they prefer after surgery is the magic of helping patients find their best outcome. Only they can truly decide, but when given clear explanations many patients choose very well, understanding it's not always an easy choice.

## Should I choose Monovision at the time of my cataract surgery?

Monovision means a person uses one eye for near vision and the other eye for distance, the goal being a clear vision in each eye for each specified focal range. Approximately 10% of patients in my experience choose monovision with their cataract surgery. Also, most surgeons do not charge extra for Monovision.

Monovision can be performed with a standard lens implant (IOL) or a Toric lens implant (corrects astigmatism, can sharpen focus), or a Light Adjustable Lens (LAL).

Monovision means a person uses one eye for distance and the other eye for near vision. During an initial consultation, a simple test is performed to determine which eye should be the distance eye for monovision. We usually start by asking each prospective patient, "Which is your shooting eye?" This usually confirms to me which eye the brain prefers for distance. Or a patient will look through a small opening to locate a target which will also determine preference. Approximately 75% of people are right eye dominant and prefer the right eye for distance, leaving the left eye better suited for near vision.

A contact lens focused on distance vision is prescribed for the dominant eye. The other eye is left nearsighted.

The brain will naturally compensate for the specific tasks and vision will be corrected and restored to a much-improved level. In a majority of cases, the patient is now glasses-free and experiencing the quality of vision of an average 30-year-old.

Today's customized eye surgery requires a better understanding of the patient's preferences, hobbies, and lifestyles. Patients who are hunters or truck drivers for example, usually prefer both eyes for distance as they require uncompromised distance vision. Other patients whose professions require less nighttime vision benefit from monovision. Usually, for those who are in academia and read or write continuously, We encourage the use of bifocals or dedicated reading glasses to accommodate their primary near vision lifestyle. Also, many patients having eye surgery with LASIK or a lens implant procedure for cataracts prefer to keep monovision after their procedure. They simply choose to discard their contacts and request their focus be surgically adjusted the way they like it.

**What Is Astigmatism?**

Astigmatism is the visual blur (without glasses) from an oval-shaped eye or cornea.

Astigmatism is important because it can cause more need for glasses after surgery than patients desire. Needing glasses for astigmatism can be reduced surgically at the time of cataract removal, more on this to come.

**What Causes Astigmatism?**

The Shape of the Eye.

(due to an oval-shaped cornea)

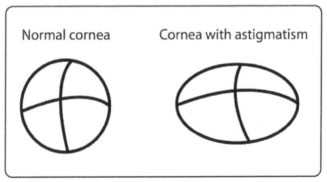

Normal cornea          Cornea with astigmatism

NIH: ttps://nei.nih.gov/health/errors/astigmatism

Many of us are born with corneas that are not round. A round cornea can make a sharp image on the macula by placing a round lens implant in the eye.

An oval-shaped cornea will produce a blurred image on the back of the retina.

Astigmatism can occur after cataract surgery and is apparent by blurred vision caused by a variance in eye shape. Round eyes produce better focus without glasses than oval-shaped eyes. The solution to astigmatism is usually an eyeglass prescription.

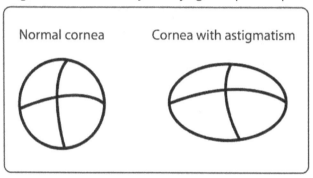

Normal cornea     Cornea with astigmatism

Some insight is gained by measuring the front surface of the eye, the cornea, using a two-dimensional map called, Topography.  A Topography Map, or "Topos" is a two-dimensional map that measures corneal steepness (think of a topography map—the terrain identified by a color code based on the height and shape of a mountain for example).

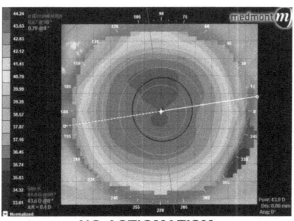

## NO ASTIGMATISM
## (Normal Topography Shown here, a 'Round' Cornea)

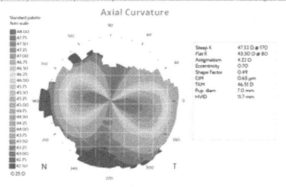

## Regular Astigmatism: It is symmetric, like a bowtie shown above in this topography measurement

Corneal Astigmatism is significant because it causes visual blurring which is then usually corrected by eyeglasses. And this can be frustrating to patients who go into cataract surgery with overly optimistic expectations. Unfortunately, people's corneas vary in shape— a determining factor in developing Astigmatism. Your friend's cornea may be round and yours may be oval. Some people have irregular corneas like the example below.

**IRREGULAR ASTIGMATISM: A less common form that can be difficult to correct unless hard contact lenses are used or more surgery is performed.**

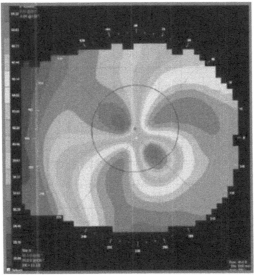

**The topography of Irregular Astigmatism**

Irregular corneas need special treatment after cataract surgery. Removing the cataract is not sufficient to enable high-functioning vision without glasses. It's just not possible. It's like looking through a half-inflated water balloon and expecting to see clearly. A corneal specialist may recommend rigid gas-permeable contact lenses or specialty surgery for the cornea.

**Should I get a Toric Lens Implant at the time of my Cataract Surgery?**

Astigmatism has a reasonable, but not perfect, chance of being corrected through a Toric Intraocular Lens Implant, or Toric IOL. Toric IOLs generally assist in reducing astigmatism. When using Toric IOLs, approximately 80% of patients achieve desired independence from glasses for a single chosen focal point—either near or distance vision.

**Should We pay extra dollars for a Femtosecond laser-assisted procedure at the time of my cataract surgery?**

Femtosecond Lasers can now assist steps of cataract surgery including incisions, capsulorhexis, nucleus segmentation, and corneal relaxing incisions for correction of astigmatism.

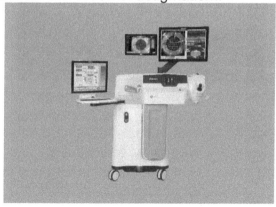

**The femtosecond laser LensX by Alcon™**

**Improving steps of surgery and the focus after surgery are potential benefits with the Femto-laser:**

**Capsulorhexis with Femto-laser**

The laser can circularly open the capsule with the laser. By creating a perfect circle that is laser-designed and centered, the centration of the lens implant may be more reliable and consistent.

**Lens segmentation with Femtolaser**

Femto-lasers are used to 'soften up' the cataract with the laser segmentation, which may allow for aspirating the nucleus with less energy.

**Astigmatism Control with Femtolaser**

One advantage of Femto-Laser Assisted Cataract Surgery (FLACS) is the arcuate corneal incisions that can reduce astigmatism. The reduction of astigmatism improves focus without glasses. By making the eye more 'round' in its shape, light rays entering the eye have a better focus on the retina, producing clearer images than if the eye was oval-shaped. Glasses are the default option for improving focus due to astigmatism, and many times, but not always, independence from glasses is improved Many studies have shown very low complication rates with either procedure. To be clear, complications occur in both groups. A surgeon's opinion of the safest approach is often his safest approach for the circumstance of the patient's condition.

Because multifocal lens implants seek as a significant goal to be less dependent on glasses, we use every option to enhance the best focus achievable, including femtosecond laser-assisted surgery. The reduction of astigmatism is a nice tool in the toolbox for achieving the best visual outcomes possible.

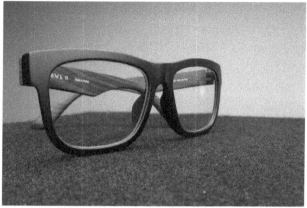

**Should We "give up near vision" for distance visual focus at the time of cataract surgery?**
A common dilemma faced by a cataract surgery patient is whether to target for "near vision" or "distance vision" because a standard lens implant will only allow for one focal point. In practical terms, a patient who chooses distance vision would no longer have a nearsighted vision without additional glasses or correction. In this sense, We try to warn patients, "Your near vision will be worse if you go for distance focus", especially to those accustomed to a lifetime of near focus or nearsightedness.
**What is Presbyopia?**

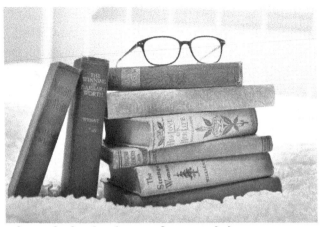

**Presbyopia is the loss of near vision or near focus due to age.**

When we are born, the lens in our eyes is usually clear for the vast majority of people. As we age, this ball of crystalline proteins becomes less pliable resulting in a gradual loss of visual range. We lose our near vision. Our "arms get longer" as we have to hold things out to read them.

The average 55-year-old is used to presbyopia because it sets in around 45 years old. A 40-year-old having cataract surgery will be more surprised that surgery with a single focus lens implant, comes with presbyopic side effects. The standard lens implant does not move or change its focal point. This is important if you are younger than 45 years old and considering cataract surgery or lens implant surgery refractive reasons.

During the initial eye consultation, we often discuss the loss of near vision is very common for humankind in their 40s and 50s. We also explain that once the human lens loses its ability to change shape, near vision is compromised and bifocals, cheater reading glasses, progressive readers, or monovision contacts are soon required to correct the deficiency. Commonly, eyeglass prescriptions offer enough "near power" compensation for reading the fine print, albeit with a progressive or bifocal aspect to the glasses. Multifocal lens implants are of course intended to overcome presbyopia and provide a depth of focus, including intermediate or near the range of vision, albeit with some compromises, including possible increased risk of night glare, halo, or visual contrast decline.

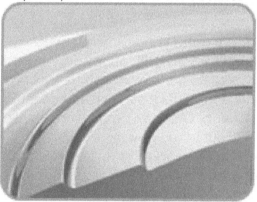

**Diffractive rings on a multifocal lens implant**
**Will We have Clear Vision without Glasses After Cataract Surgery?**
That depends on your goals and definition of improvement. There are many factors, mostly need for glasses is a common goal that is not yet perfected for all patients. You may need glasses. The shape of eyes varies amongst patients, and this affects the outcome of focus that patients may

discuss.  Factors for refractive satisfaction include: is the eye is round vs. oval-shaped (astigmatic), which lens did you choose, the patient's eye health, your visual needs, and willingness to get by without glasses.

Some patients are of low maintenance.  "Just give me glasses after surgery. We will wear them 100% of the time. We just want the cataract removed." They are the easiest to please in terms of focus. They expect glasses and are okay with that. A standard monofocal lens implant usually satisfies this low bar of visual need for this request.

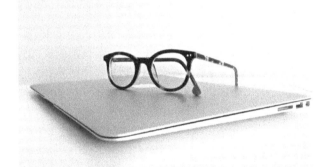

Given the choice, many patients prefer a clearer uncorrected vision without glasses. Modern intraocular lenses have an improving success rate in obtaining good uncorrected vision for the visual range of the patient's choice, yet we seek better results all the time.

**The following categories provide a general composite of potential cataract surgery patient's goals.  Understanding your visual needs and**

**hopes will help guide your decision-making for lens type and decisions with your surgeon.**

**Distance** Seekers. "Good distance with both eyes without glasses is my hope. We will wear reading glasses for all near activities - like reading, doing make-up, tying fishing lures, etc.."

Usually, a standard lens implant, or a Toric lens implant if necessary, can assist to target this goal. Probably 65% of my patients fall into this category.

**Near** Seekers. "Good near vision without glasses with both eyes is fine. We love to sew & read, and hope to do so without glasses. We will wear glasses for distance, television, driving, and outdoors."

Usually, a standard lens implant, or a Toric lens implant if necessary, can assist to target this goal. Probably 15% of my patients fall into this category.

**Monovision.** "We like one eye set for near vision and one eye set for distance vision. I've done this with contact lenses and it works great. We often use glasses for night driving or reading novels because the compromise causes strain at those times."

Usually, a standard lens implant, or a Toric lens implant if necessary, can assist to target this goal. Probably 10% of my patients fall into this category.

**Distance & Near** Seekers. "Good distance with both eyes without glasses is my hope. We would like near vision if possible and We want the balance of both eyes being the same focus (not monovision). We will wear glasses if We have to do so, perhaps for very near activities like tying fishing lures or small print.

Usually, a **Multifocal** lens implant, with or without additional astigmatism correction, can assist to target this goal. Probably 10% of my patients fall into this category due to the increased cost of such lens implants and the suitability or risks of these lenses.

**the Restor Multifocal lens implant**

Choosing cataract surgery provides a unique opportunity to improve on one or more of the above goals. Through this procedure, chances are your vision will improve. The question remains, however: Will this surgery fail, meet, or exceed your expectations? It often depends on what you expect, hence a good discussion with your ophthalmologist will clarity your suitability.

**Panoptix Trifocal Lens Implant by Alcon, FDA approved in 2019 in the U.S.**

The first FDA-approved Trifocal lens implant in the United States was approved in 2019, the **Panoptix** multifocal IOL by Alcon. Panoptix is designed to target all three zones of functional vision focal length: distance focus, mid-range (about 20 inches from one's eyes or laptop distance typically), and near focus (15 inches from your eyes, e.g. book reading or small print).

The **Panoptix** utilizes diffraction. Light is split by the lens implant into 3 focal points inside the eye, and an object to be visualized is brought closer to the focus of the patient, an image is produced by the lens to focus on the back of the eye or the macula. The functionality of a trifocal lens implant for those seeking to be less dependent on spectacles is improving generally with newer generations of lens multifocal lenses. Our first ReStor We placed in residency in 2006, and now a decade and a half later we have better range, less unwanted halos and glare at night, and improving equipment to control and treat astigmatism and focus.

10% to 20% of patients, unfortunately, will probably require some glasses use despite having a multifocal lens implant placed. It's a constant hope and ambition to meet the expectations of patients, but risks of requiring glasses exist. Even in uncomplicated situations, glasses may still be required.

**Refractive Outcome Improvements by Measuring Technology:**

Fortunately, Zeiss has issued a new measuring device that in my experience has improved our outcomes and chances of controlling astigmatism and improving the focus for patients after surgery. Also, the LensX laser assists to standardize the size of the capsulorhexis during surgery and perform laser corneal incisions that relax astigmatism. These contributions enhance options for the surgeon and nudge the focus outcomes to sharper focus in a beneficial way for patients.

**Financial Cost**

The additional costs for these technologies pose a barrier for some patients to get access. While it's ideal to have a range of vision unaided from spectacles, not all patients can afford it. Typically insurance will not cover the allowable extra costs for these elective focus procedures of astigmatism control and a multi-focal presbyopic lens implant. Not all patients may be ideal candidates or may desire to choose a multifocal lens, such as if the eye has factors of additional conditions or eye disease that may adversely affect the performance of the presbyopic IOL. If a patient is in a low vision situation, and the cataract is only a part of their visual decline, then a standard lens implant and glasses may be more medically indicated to assist recovery of vision.

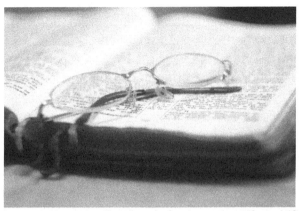

Glasses are generally the default option if multifocal lens implants are unable to reduce the dependence on glasses. While it may be expensive to do multifocal lenses, seek astigmatism correction, and then still utilize glasses, there is simply no guarantee a person will never require glasses for distance, or near, or both. Generally, the percentages are favorable and many patients are pleased to reduce glasses dependence by multi-focal lens implants and femtosecond laser-assisted cataract surgery (FLACS).

**What eye drops will We be prescribed after cataract surgery?**

For patients with no drug allergies, we typically place antibiotics inside the eye after surgery, and no prescribed eye drop antibiotics are done. For those with allergies to quinolones (Ciprofloxacin, Levofloxacin (Levaquin), Moxifloxacin, or Ofloxacin), We typically prescribe an antibiotic drop four times daily for ten days in a different category. We usually prescribe an anti-inflammatory eye drop for ten days (NSAIDs). A steroid injection of Triamcinolone or

Kenalog is done under the conjunctiva with the cataract surgery or a Prednisolone steroid drop for 30 days. These collective prescriptive medications promote good healing and are important in preventing infection, inflammation, and swelling.

**Will my Cataract Surgery be a Success?**

"If you don't know where you are going, you will wind up somewhere else."

Yogi Berra

What factors determine successful cataract surgery? One obvious factor would include empirical evidence. Most patients feel they have undergone successful surgery if they see better than they did before. There are some patients however who have such high expectations that any variation of outcome (when compared to their peers) sets them back emotionally. Yes, they can see better than before but not as well as they thought they would. Therefore, patients must be realistic in both expectations and outcomes. Again, there are many factors to consider when opting for cataract surgery and those factors often determine the level and quality of success. Eye shape, the degree of visual correction, dry eyes, macular disease, the shape of the cornea, and astigmatism are just a few examples. Additional factors may include the patient's visual preference, personality, lifestyle, habits, and activities.

Therefore the discussion of these factors between doctor and patient is vital in determining whether or not a patient is a good candidate for cataract surgery and if so, what the patient can reasonably expect from such surgery.

**Special Situations:  Cataract Surgery after LASIK surgery**

**Post LASIK cataract surgery:  sharpening the focus**

At least 20 different formulas have been published about how to calculate Lens Implant power for the post-LASIK patient.  Measurement devices approximate the lens implant power, but central corneal changes from LASIK influence final focus outcomes in a manner not entirely measured.  The American Society of Cataract & Refractive Surgery assists surgeons on a free basis for IOL measurements in these cases with an online calculator tool to approximate as many methods as currently available data for each patient will allow. Each surgeon develops a technique of their comfort and experience to approach refractive accuracy.
 Ultimately, improving technology aids outcomes.  In many cases, the best data available from prior LASIK enables better calculations of focus after cataract surgery

**What are the risks & complications of cataract surgery?**

Unexpected complications may include Infection in the eye (endophthalmitis); retinal detachment; a retained cataract; inflammation; Glaucoma (high eye pressure causing damage to the optic nerve); a broken capsular bag (which can cause difficulty in placing the intraocular lens implant); chronic floaters; an increased edge glare or glare from store lights, bothersome 'twinkle' in the eye as seen in photos, and other concerns.

**What is the risk of retinal detachment?**

Retinal detachments occur when the nerve tissue (the retina) inside the eye (which works like the 'film in the camera' of the eye) gets torn or becomes detached. Though relatively rare, retinal detachments can cause devastating visual loss.

In many cases, it can occur without any surgery but can also occur after surgery as well. If the retina can be layered or operated on before the macula (or central part of the retina) is involved in the detachment, then the prognosis is usually better than if the macula is detached. Vision loss occurs when a detached retina causes injury to important cells in the retina.

Many methods are utilized by a retinal specialist to reattach a detached retina, the most common being the surgical removal of the vitreous gel in the back of the eye (vitrectomy) and the draining of fluid from behind the retina. Then, endolaser laser treatment is used to help seal down the retinal breaks, holes, or tears that led to the detachment.

Other common options include using gas or oil to fill the eye over days, weeks, or even months to rehabilitate the attachment of the laser to the inside wall of the eye (choroid). Also, a band of plastic or silicone can be placed surgically around the eye like a belt (a scleral buckle), changing vector forces and allowing the retina much better conformity to be reattached and prevent recurrence of the retinal detachment.

**What is the Risk of Infection in the eye?**
The estimated rate of infection inside the eye (called 'endophthalmitis') is rare, occurring approximately one per every 3000 cases. This low rate of infection is due primarily to the use of smaller incisions and the avoidance of sutures which can commonly be a source for infection. Paradoxically, We place a suture in any wound that does not demonstrate watertight closure, to avoid leak and infection. Bacteria entering the eye through a leaky wound after surgery is most likely the cause of rare endophthalmitis.

**The rare case of endopthalmitis can be devastating and cause vision loss.**
Endophthalmitis occurs when bacteria infiltrate the inside of the eye and start to grow, causing inflammation, damage, and eventual loss of vision. In these cases, prompt treatment is vital in saving and restoring the eye and its vision. Due to the nature of the surgery, however, even strict guidelines and care measures cannot guarantee a 100% prevention rate.

**What is the risk of Retained Cataract Fragment?**
Although uncommon, even the best surgeons must occasionally return to the operating room to retrieve a small piece of cataract left behind during the initial cataract surgery. These small pieces are sometimes trapped under the iris and are thus unable to be removed by the vacuum devices used during surgery (phacoemulsification). Retained cataract fragments can cause elevated eye pressure (glaucoma), inflammation, and other undesired

consequences. In such cases, a physician and patient can choose to either wait it out (if the inflammation and eye pressure elevation are controllable with drops) or return to surgery.

## What is the risk of a broken posterior capsule during surgery?

A broken capsular bag during cataract surgery is rare. Nevertheless, it is a surgical risk that all surgeons and patients must take into account.

 The risks become greater when placing a lens implant and those risks increase in cases where glaucoma, inflammation, and retinal detachment are present. Occasionally, a lens implant can still be placed inside the capsular bag or just in front of the capsular bag (in the ciliary sulcus). Clean-up of vitreous gel protruding through the capsular bag (anterior vitrectomy) may be required in such cases. If the capsular bag is disrupted to a certain degree, then a lens implant must either be sutured in place (scleral sutured IOL) or placed in the front chamber of the eye (Anterior Chamber IOL).

## What is PCO and how is it treated?

PCO stands for "Posterior Capsular Opacity." The capsular bag holding the lens implant eventually becomes cloudy after cataract surgery. This is a relatively common condition, usually occurring earlier in life for younger healthier patients, and its rate of development can vary from a few months to many years.

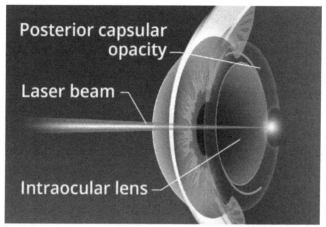

**Yag laser capsulotomy opening the posterior capsule sometime later after cataract surgery**

Eventually, almost all patients who have had cataract surgery will develop a cloudy haze (PCO) that affects their vision (this condition occurs inside the capsular bag that holds the intraocular lens implant (IOL).

The need for PCO treatment can occur months or even years after surgery, even when the capsule is meticulously cleaned at the time of surgery.

**Posterior Capsular Opacification (PCO) may require Yag Laser Capsulotomy**

Treatment for PCO is performed by using a laser that creates an opening in the posterior capsule, improving the visual haze. When the posterior capsule is opened, the vision typically improves as the pathway for light is now less obstructed.

The risks of using a YAG laser to treat PCO include the presence of new floaters in one's vision; worse floaters; and on rare occasions, retinal tears, retinal detachments, or complete loss of vision. Increased or continued glare after the use of a Yag laser is also a risk.

**What are the risks of prior LASIK for Cataract Surgery Patients?**

LASIK is a procedure to refocus the eye by using a to change corneal shape. Even with additional measurements and additional calculations, Post-LASIK patients have a cornea that's been altered, making it less favorable for predictable visual focus outcomes. Needing glasses is a risk of surgery, even with the most sophisticated measuring devices. Having available prior LASIK data helps adjust these calculations and accuracy. Having comparative data from prior LASIK surgery enables improved optimization of visual outcomes with adjustments to calculations from current corneal measurements.

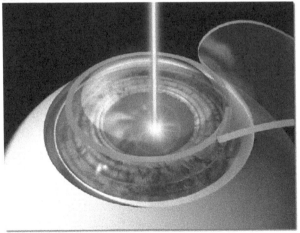

Because LASIK surgery changes the shape of the front of the cornea, routine measuring instruments for lens implant power can become less accurate based on the post-refractive corneal shape. The development of new technology, however, has improved the success rate of calculating IOL power in LASIK surgery patients. Many formulas are available to cataract surgeons to optimize visual targets for the patient who had LASIK in the past. Many times, simply knowing a patient's glasses prescription before and after LASIK surgery, allows for proper focal adjustment. Estimates can be made for patients who do not know their glasses prescription before LASIK surgery. Such estimation can be accomplished by knowing the patient's history and current measurements of corneal shape as well as their prior contact lens prescriptions. The direct and exact measurement of corneal power is tricky because these corneas are often multifocal. In other words, the focus of the cornea is not uniform after LASIK and can result in a "multifocal" type focus, increasing ambiguity in measurements. We have had success using the Post LASIK calculator offered by ASCRS (American Society of Cataract & Refractive Surgery). When no prior data is provided, We interview my patients in-depth to determine their medical history to estimate the correct power.

We also use the Topography measurements of the patient to estimate the type of LASIK performed and the degree of diopters possibly treated by looking at peripheral to central corneal shape.

Surgeon-to-patient communication is key to improving a patient's understanding of the risks and benefits of LASIK surgery. The use of Multifocal

Lens Implants that require precise focus after surgery is perhaps asking a bit much of today's technology. Multifocal lens implants are categorized as "off-label" by the FDA since the FDA did not observe trial study patients when approving them for general use. So even though they can be prescribed, there are potential risks associated with their use.

**What are the risks of prior RK (Radial Keratotomy) for cataract surgery patients?**
Radial Keratotomy or "RK" (making incisions in the cornea) was first utilized in the 1980s and early 1990s to correct nearsightedness. RK has been shown to have some downsides however so it is generally not performed anymore in the U.S.

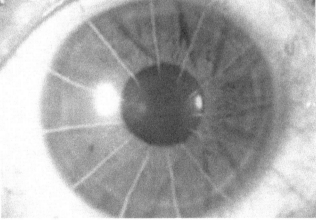

**Radial Keratotomy Corneal Incisions are done to Treat Myopia as a Refractive Procedure**
Radial Keratotomy patients have a corneal shape that can affect their visual focus after surgery. Because of this condition, their vision may fluctuate to a greater degree than average a month or two

after surgery. These patients may have long-term daily fluctuation in their vision and may even become more farsighted over months or even years.

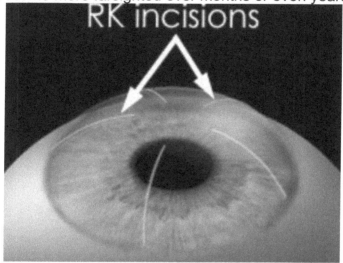

**RK can affect visual outcomes after cataract surgery**

**What are common eye drop regimens like after surgery?**

Injections are more commonly being done to reduce the need for eye drops after surgery, making recovery more comfortable, while also protecting from infection and inflammation after surgery. Typically an injection of antibiotics and a steroid (for anti-inflammatory purposes) are utilized.

Non-steroid anti-inflammatory (NSAID) eye drops also protect from complications of swelling in the macula after cataract surgery and are utilized for several days or weeks after surgery. Typically the NSAID drops are started 1-2 days before surgery and continue after surgery. Diabetics begin the eye drops 1 week before surgery. NSAID can be prescribed once (Ilevro or Prolensa) or twice daily (generic ketoralac drops). After several weeks of use of the generic ketorolac, the chance of irritation and dry eye symptoms, and blurry vision rises, so limiting to a few weeks is preferred when possible.

**What is Glaucoma?**

Glaucoma is a condition of increasing damage and subsequent vision loss due to optic nerve fiber cell death. As optic nerve fibers deteriorate, the process of damage may be slowed down or halted by lowering the eye pressure. Intraocular pressure (IOP) is measured to determine the risk of glaucoma damage to advance. The high pressure causes an increased risk of glaucoma damage. In some cases of uncontrolled glaucoma, (or sometimes quickly with sudden high pressure), vision is lost over time.

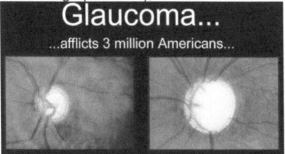

**Optic nerve damage and excavation in glaucoma**

Glaucoma can be detected and treated in most cases with an eye exam that measures eye pressure and examines the optic nerve. A damaged optic nerve appears to have glaucoma if it has a thinned rim of nerve fiber tissue. This can be observed by a physician in many cases and measured with optic nerve scans using ultrasound, called an OCT scan (optical coherence tonometry). OCT has become a more common clinical test and frequently used for diagnosis and monitoring of glaucoma progression.

Some clinical tests will help confirm diagnosis such as measurements of peripheral vision and measurements of the OCT imaging.

**Can glaucoma be controlled by surgery at the same time as my cataract surgery?**

Many patients with cataracts also develop glaucoma. The onset of both conditions more frequently occurs after the age of fifty.

Cataract surgery may be combined with other procedures that lower eye pressure, including endocylophotocoagulation (ECP), Goniotomy, Trabecular micro-bypass stent implantation, Hydrus trabecular stent, and other procedures.

Glaucoma may be controlled with topical eye drop medications prescribed by your eye doctor, by laser treatment to the trabecular meshwork or the ciliary body, and by stenting procedures that shunt aqueous out of the eye to areas of lower pressure. Such stents or shunts include Xen glaucoma stents to the subconjunctival space, glaucoma tube shunt procedures, and filtration surgery such as by an Xpress scleral implant filtration device to a scleral flap and conjunctival bleb.

Typically, the least invasive procedure with a reduction of pressure is advised that it can successfully control eye pressure and limit glaucoma progression. For advanced glaucoma situations, a more significant procedure may be indicated to help reduce the risk of further glaucoma damage. Consulting with a physician experienced in the spectrum of glaucoma surgeries can guide your decision-making.

**Does Cataract Surgery lower eye pressure?**
Many studies have shown the benefits of cataract-removal to lower eye pressure. Intraocular pressure is lowered by several points (mm of mercury) and may be more effective in lowering eye pressure in cases of narrow-angle anatomy inside the eye.

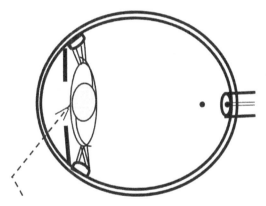

**INTRAOCULAR LENS IMPLANT (IOL)**

Space in the anterior chamber is increased with the removal of the cataract and placement of the intraocular lens implant. The IOL is thinner than the human lens. The iris rests back with the removal of the cataractous lens. This likely benefits intraocular pressure as the angle from the iris to the cornea is widened, allowing the drainage angle more space and facilitating aqueous drainage and lower intraocular pressure.

**Trabecular Stent for Glaucoma at the time of Cataract Surgery:    IStent by Glaucos**

The iStent by Glaucos is a micro-invasive glaucoma device and one of the first such devices to use a stent from inside the "angle" of the eye. We have used the iStent in my practice since 2014. (We often use eye drops in conjunction with the iStent due to the overall pressure-lowering effect).

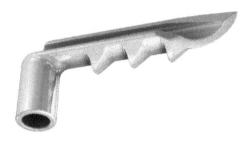

**the iStent**

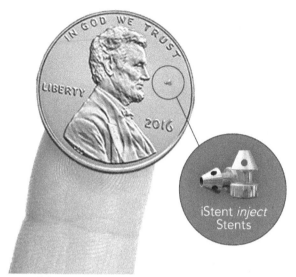

**Size of the iStent inject stents**

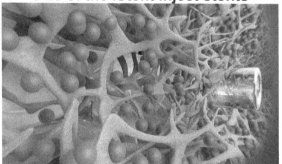

**An iStent depicted implanted in the Trabecular Meshwork of Schlemm's canal**

The iStent is placed through the drainage resistance barrier called the Trabecular Meshwork (TM). The iStent allows the flow of aqueous through the TM into the Schlemm's canal, where natural drainage occurs, into collector channels that carry this fluid away from and outside the eye. IStent can be combined with cataract surgery and ECP to increase the effectiveness in lowering eye pressure. The iStent is approved exclusively through Medicare in the United States and prescribed for patients with mild to moderate glaucoma.

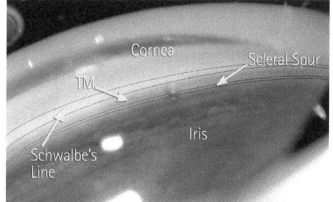

**An iStent shown implanted in Schlemm's canal**

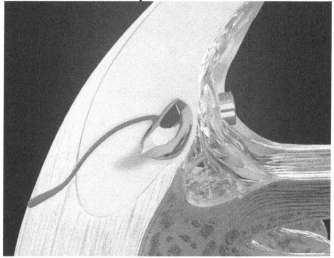

**iStent implanted in Trabecular Meshwork of the drainage angle of the eye**

## Hydrus Glaucoma Trabecular Bypass Stent by Ivantis

Hydrus is a micro-stent placed by the surgeon in Schlemm's canal via a canalotomy. It functions to stretch the trabecular meshwork and increase flow into the collector system to lower intraocular pressure.

Here is an accurate appraisal by Google:

'This minimally invasive technique, the Hydrus stent is highly effective in reducing the pressure in those with glaucoma. The technique has been shown in studies to reduce the need for taking glaucoma drops and the majority of patients are off drops altogether.

The Hydrus® Microstent is an implantable, flexible, metal (nitinol) tube with windows (open-back stent) pre-loaded onto a hand-held delivery system. Sep 14, 2018 Studies have found the Hydrus to be very safe for those who qualify for the surgery. How does the Hydrus work? The Hydrus device is made of a tiny tube. The Hydrus creates a path that allows the fluid inside the eye to bypass the natural drain of the eye.

Because this is a minimally invasive procedure, the risk of complications is low. In some cases, there is a small bleed in the eye that resolves within a week. On rare occasions, the eye pressure can rise for a few days after surgery, but this can be treated effectively with additional eye drops.'

## Glaucoma Surgery at the time of Cataract Surgery:

## ECP:  Endocyclophotocoagulation

Endocyclophotocoagulation (ECP) is a laser procedure performed on the ciliary body, an area in the eye that produces fluid inside the eye (aqueous humor).

Eye pressure is determined by the production and drainage of this aqueous fluid inside the eye. ECP lowers eye pressure, a useful treatment for glaucoma. ECP can also be used for many types of glaucoma including most types of open-angle glaucoma and angle-closure glaucoma and its side effect profile is favorable in most cases. Side effects can include increased inflammation inside the eye which is often treated with topical anti-inflammatory eye drops after surgery in a similar fashion to non-ECP cataract surgery cases.

**ECP and Cataract removal for Narrow Angle Glaucoma**

Cataract and ECP laser are particularly effective in treating a type of glaucoma known as narrow-angle glaucoma. Narrow-angle glaucoma is a collapse or blockage of the iris and cornea where the anatomic angle leads to the drainage canal of the eye, Schlemm's canal.

**Glaucoma Surgery at the time of Cataract Surgery:**

**Goniotomy**

A **goniotomy** is an eye pressure-lowering procedure that opens or incises the area of resistance to drainage of flow out of the eye, called the Trabecular Meshwork. Goniotomy can be performed during cataract surgery with a Kahook Dual Blade (KDB) or other devices. Goniotomy can be used in childhood glaucoma, a much less common condition than glaucoma in adults. Due to the increasing development of methods for performing goniotomy, its practice may become standard in the future. As of now, glaucoma specialists and some cataract surgeons utilize goniotomy on a relatively frequent basis. Instruments to perform goniotomy have become more refined for 2022. New World Medical has just launched an improved instrument the KDB-Glide. It's smaller and easier to use in the canal to open the trabecular meshwork than the previous original Kahook Dual Blade device. Another iteration is now available for washing out the canal (viscodilation) and goniotomy simultaneously. The Omni device was the original pioneer procedure which allowed surgeons to perform these tasks, and is still available. A new device in 2022 is the Streamline Goniotomy by New World Medical. It performs 7 small goniotomies and is able to flush Schlemm's canal with a viscoelastic material. Data on it's efficacy is pending. It may have significnat advantages for patients on blood-thinners, such as Coumadin, Warfarin, Lovenox, or Eliquis. The smaller goniotomies are less likely to reflux red blood cells into the anterior chamber of they eye, an incremental improvement in safety for goniotomy given it is one of the risks for the KDB GLIDE goniotomy procedure.

**Glaucoma Surgery Options**
**Filtration Procedures: shunt aqueous out of the eye**

Filtration procedures lower eye pressure by allowing fluid out of the front chamber of the eye to the space outside the eye. This can be done with a surgically made tunnel under a scleral flap (trabeculectomy), by a silicone catheter to a reservoir (Baerveldt or Ahmed Glaucoma drainage tube, or placing a shunt device in the eye (Xpress shunt, or Xen stent). Patients requiring filtration surgery have poorly controlled or advanced glaucoma, and a typically higher risk of vision loss from their glaucoma. More significant reductions in pressure are achieved with filtration surgery and often can reduce the use of medications.

**XEN**

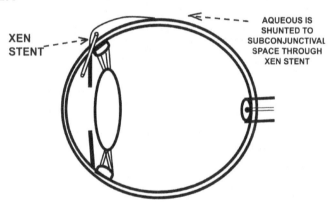

XEN STENT

AQUEOUS IS SHUNTED TO SUBCONJUNCTIVAL SPACE THROUGH XEN STENT

**XEN GEL STENT ACCESS THE ANTERIOR CHAMBER TO DRAIN AQUEOUS TO SUBCONJUNCTIVAL SPACE**

**XEN® Stent by Allergan**

Xen stents have been in use since 2016. Xen stents may be placed from an internal approach through a corneal incision, or an external approach by passing through conjunctiva and sclera externally.

# Glaucoma Tube shunt - Baerveldt, Ahmed, & Ahmed Clearpath

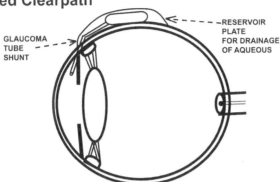

**GLAUCOMA TUBE SHUNTS ACCESS THE ANTERIOR CHAMBER TO DRAIN AQUEOUS**

Baerveldt glaucoma drainage tube surgery is generally reserved for a standalone procedure (not at the same time as cataract surgery) but may be combined with cataract surgery. Glaucoma tube shunts may be done for glaucoma control for neovascular glaucoma, or cases where other glaucoma surgeries are more likely to fail and scar down and lose filtration.

**Xpress Filtration Procedure**

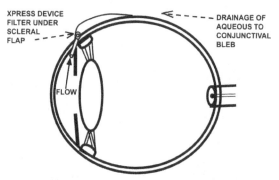

**XPRESS DEVICE UNDER SCLERAL FLAP**
DRAIN AQUEOUS TO SUBCONJUNCTIVAL SPACE

An Xpress implant placed beneath a scleral flap enables drainage to a subconjunctival bleb to lower intraocular pressure. The advantage of the Xpress is to place a device that will control flow and remove scarring for flow at the site of its implantation. The conjunctival bleb is formed from aqueous flowing beneath the scleral flap.

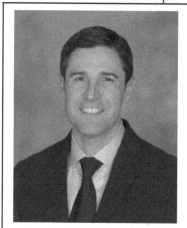

David Woods, MD

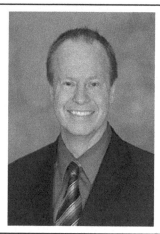

Robert B. Reeve, MD

Chico, California
w ww.ReeveWoods.com
Cataract, Laser, & Glaucoma Surgery

**Cataract Surgery Expertise**

Patients with cataracts have more options available now than ever before. By performing standard cataract surgery, custom cataract surgery with multifocal lens implants, or correcting astigmatism at the time of cataract surgery, patients have an array of options to fit their visual lifestyle.

**Dr. David Woods, MD**

**Licensure & Training:** University of Washington School of Medicine, Seattle WA

**Externship:** All-India Institute of Medical Sciences, Delhi, India, 2002

**Internship:** University of Washington at Boise, VAMC Hospital, 2003

**Residency:** UC Davis Department of Ophthalmology, Sacramento CA. 2003 - 2006

**Board Certification:** American Board of Ophthalmology, 2008

**Practice:** Reeve Woods Eye Center, Chico CA 2006 - present

Eye Consultations, & Cataract Surgery Vision Correction

Board Certified by the American Board of Ophthalmology, Dr. Woods provides comprehensive consultations for eye disease, expertise in cataract surgery, with vision correction and glaucoma eye care. With a focus on safety and reducing the risks of surgery, Dr. Woods explains the evidence of eye problems, medical or surgical treatment options, and answer questions you may have about your eyes or vision. Using high-quality surgical and medical techniques, and focusing on patient-oriented care with custom visual outcomes, Dr. Woods aims to provide the safest possible care for your eye procedure.

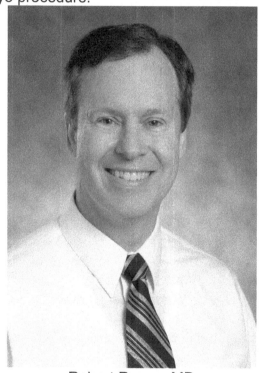

Robert Reeve, MD
Eye Care Physician & Surgeon
Chico & Paradise, California
Www.ReeveWoods.com
Cataract, Laser, & Glaucoma Surgery

**Education:**

**Licensure & Training:** University of Utah School of Medicine, Salt Lake City, UT
**Internship:** University of Michigan, Ann Arbor
**Residency:** University of Michigan, Ann Arbor
**Fellowship:** University of Michigan, Ann Arbor
**Board Certification:** American Board of Ophthalmology,
**Practice:** Reeve Woods Eye Center, Chico CA
**Quality Eye Care and a Commitment to Safety**
Make your eye care a comfortable and informative experience. By answering questions, and a commitment to reducing surgical risks with a patient-centered approach, Dr. Woods and Dr. Reeve have performed tens of thousands of eye procedures in Northern California. Their office is located in Chico, California at Reeve Woods Eye Center.

**Schedule an Appointment**
**Reeve Woods Eye Center**
Www.ReeveWoods.com
**530-899-2244**
280 Cohasset Road
Chico, CA 95926

Made in USA - Kendallville, IN
85224_9781980526537
08.30.2022 1418